DOMINIC SINGH

Transform 360: Bariatric Surgery for a New You

A Guide to Weightloss and Incredible Health

Contents

Preface

Embarking on bariatric surgery is a life-changing decision filled with hope and determination. For many, this surgery offers a new beginning, relieving the physical and emotional burdens of obesity. However, unexpected challenges can arise.

My own journey was one of triumph and tribulation. I vividly remember the mix of excitement and anxiety as I prepared for the operation, hopeful for a healthier future. While the surgery was successful, my path soon took a harrowing turn. One of the clamps used to stitch the stomach gave way, causing excruciating pain and requiring a stent to be placed in my esophagus. For a month, I lived with this, a constant reminder of the fragility of my condition.

Those weeks were incredibly challenging, both physically and emotionally. I grappled with fear and frustration, wondering if I would ever regain my strength. However, this experience revealed a well of resilience within me and a determination to thrive.

This book is born from that realization. It is a guide and a source of comfort for anyone considering or undergoing bariatric surgery. I use my personal story as my experience alongside practical advice, expert insights, and emotional support. My hope is that this book will empower you and remind you that you are not alone.

To those considering bariatric surgery, your struggles and fears are valid, and your courage is immense. This journey is not easy, but it is one of the most rewarding paths you can take. Together, we can navigate the challenges and celebrate the victories.

With empathy and encouragement,

Dominic Singh

1

Introduction

Welcome to "Transform 360: Bariatric Surgery For A New You" This book is designed to be your comprehensive companion as you navigate the journey of bariatric surgery and embrace the transformative changes it brings to your life. Whether you're considering bariatric surgery, preparing for the procedure, or have already undergone surgery, this guide is here to provide you with essential information, practical advice, and heartfelt support every step of the way.

In the pages that follow, we'll embark on a journey together, starting with a deep dive into the world of bariatric surgery. We'll explore what bariatric surgery is, the different types of procedures available, and who may be a suitable candidate for surgery. But before we delve into the surgical aspects, we'll first lay the groundwork by understanding the complexities of obesity – its definitions, causes, and the significant health risks it poses.

From there, we'll journey through the evolution of bariatric surgery, tracing its historical roots, celebrating its remarkable advancements, and looking ahead to the promising future of weight loss interventions. We'll then guide you through the crucial process of preparing for surgery, covering everything from preoperative evaluations to the essential dietary and lifestyle changes needed to optimize your health before surgery. Additionally, we'll delve into the importance of psychological preparation and address financial considerations to ensure you're fully equipped for this transformative journey.

Once you're ready, we'll walk you through the surgical process itself, offering a comprehensive overview of what to expect before, during, and after surgery. We'll provide insights into hospital stays, recovery periods, and postoperative care, empowering you with the knowledge needed to navigate this critical phase with confidence.

But our journey doesn't end there. It's only just beginning. We'll then shift our focus to life after bariatric surgery, exploring the dietary guidelines, nutritional strategies, and exercise recommendations necessary for long-term success. We'll delve into the emotional and psychological changes that often accompany weight loss, offering practical advice and support for managing these transitions. We'll equip you with strategies for addressing and overcoming potential complications and side effects, ensuring you have the tools needed to navigate any challenges that may arise.

Through it all, we share all the triumph and resilience, offering inspiration and encouragement as you embark on your journey of transformation. From setting goals to overcoming obstacles, we stand by your side, offering support and guidance every step of the way.

So, whether you're just beginning to explore the possibility of bariatric surgery or are already on your postoperative journey, know that you're not alone. "A Guide to Bariatric Surgery and Life Beyond" is more than just a book—it's a road map to a healthier, happier future. Whether you're considering bariatric surgery for yourself or supporting a loved one through the process, this guide is your comprehensive resource for understanding, preparing for, and thriving after bariatric surgery. Together, let's embark on this transformative journey towards a healthier, happier you.

2

Understanding Bariatric Surgery

What is Bariatric Surgery?

Bariatric surgery, often referred to as weight-loss surgery or metabolic surgery, is a medical procedure performed on the stomach or intestines to aid in weight loss for individuals who are severely obese. This type of surgery is typically considered when other methods of weight loss, such as diet and exercise, have not been effective or when obesity-related health conditions are particularly severe.

The most common type of bariatric surgery is gastric bypass, although there are other procedures like sleeve gastrectomy and gastric banding. These surgeries work by either restricting the amount of food the stomach can hold, reducing calorie absorption, or a combination of both. For example, gastric bypass involves creating a small pouch at the top of the stomach and connecting it directly to the small intestine, bypassing a portion of the stomach and upper intestine to reduce both the amount of food that can be eaten and the absorption of calories.

One of the significant benefits of bariatric surgery is its potential to lead to significant weight loss and improvements or resolutions of various obesity-related health problems such as type 2 diabetes, high blood pressure, and sleep apnea. Many individuals who undergo bariatric surgery experience dramatic improvements in their overall health and quality of life.

However, it's essential to recognize that bariatric surgery is not a standalone solution. Long-term success requires making permanent healthy changes to one's diet and lifestyle. Patients must adhere to dietary guidelines provided by healthcare professionals, focusing on nutrient-dense foods and portion control. Regular exercise is also crucial for maintaining weight loss, improving physical fitness, and supporting overall health.

Additionally, ongoing medical follow-up is necessary to monitor progress, address any potential complications, and provide support throughout the post-surgery journey. By combining bariatric surgery with permanent lifestyle changes and ongoing medical care, individuals can achieve long-term success in managing their weight and improving their health.

Types of Bariatric Procedures

Sleeve Gastrectomy, Roux-en-Y Gastric Bypass, Adjustable Gastric Band, Biliopancreatic Diversion with Duodenal Switch, Single Anastomosis Duodeno-Ileal Bypass with Sleeve Gastrectomy are all the procedures normally done in a Bariatric surgery.

Sleeve Gastrectomy

The Sleeve Gastrectomy, often referred to simply as the "sleeve," is a popular bariatric surgical procedure designed to assist individuals in achieving significant weight loss and improving metabolic health. During the surgery, approximately 80% of the stomach is surgically removed, resulting in a tubular or sleeve-shaped stomach resembling a banana. This reduction in stomach size restricts the amount of food and liquid that can be consumed, leading to decreased calorie intake and subsequent weight loss. By eliminating the portion of the stomach responsible for producing ghrelin, the hormone that stimulates hunger, the sleeve gastrectomy also helps to decrease feelings of hunger and promote satiety, supporting long-term weight management.

Moreover, the metabolic changes induced by the sleeve gastrectomy contribute to improved blood sugar control, making it an effective treatment option for individuals with obesity-related conditions such as type 2 diabetes. Compared to other bariatric surgeries involving manipulation of the small intestine, such as gastric bypass, sleeve gastrectomy is considered a safer and less complex procedure with a lower risk of complications. Its laparoscopic approach, utilizing small incisions and specialized instruments, minimizes surgical trauma and facilitates quicker recovery times, allowing patients to resume normal activities sooner following surgery.

However, while the sleeve gastrectomy offers significant benefits in terms of weight loss and metabolic improvement, its success ultimately depends on the individual's commitment to making permanent lifestyle changes. Following surgery, patients must adhere to dietary guidelines, engage in regular physical activity, and attend follow-up appointments with healthcare providers to monitor progress and address any post-operative issues. With dedication to these lifestyle modifications, individuals undergoing sleeve gastrectomy can achieve substantial and sustainable weight loss, leading to improved overall health and quality of life.

Roux-en-Y Gastric Bypass

The Roux-en-Y Gastric Bypass, commonly known as the "gastric bypass," is among the most frequently performed operations for treating obesity and related health conditions. Its name originates from the French term "in the form of a Y," reflecting the shape of the intestinal reconstruction involved.

During the procedure, the stomach is partitioned into a smaller upper portion, roughly the size of an egg, while the larger portion is bypassed, no longer involved in food storage or digestion. The small intestine is also divided and reconnected to the new stomach pouch, creating a bypass of the majority of the stomach and the first portion of the small intestine. This results in a gastrointestinal configuration resembling the letter Y.

The gastric bypass exerts its effects through several mechanisms. The smaller stomach pouch restricts food intake, leading to reduced calorie consumption. Additionally, by bypassing the initial portion of the small intestine where nutrient absorption primarily occurs, the procedure reduces the absorption of calories and nutrients. Importantly, the altered route of food through the gastrointestinal tract influences hormonal and metabolic processes, decreasing hunger, increasing feelings of fullness, and facilitating weight loss and maintenance. Furthermore, gastric bypass often yields improvements in metabolic health, including the resolution or improvement of conditions like adult-onset diabetes and reflux (heartburn). However, to optimize outcomes, patients must adhere to dietary guidelines, avoid certain substances like tobacco and NSAIDs, and make appropriate lifestyle choices in conjunction with the surgery.

Adjustable Gastric Band

The Adjustable Gastric Band, composed of silicone, is positioned around the upper portion of the stomach to restrict food intake. Its effectiveness in addressing obesity-related diseases and facilitating long-term weight loss falls short compared to other bariatric procedures, leading to a decline in its usage over the past decade.

During the procedure, the band is placed and secured around the upper stomach, creating a small pouch above it. The sensation of fullness relies on the size of the opening between this pouch and the remainder of the stomach, which can be adjusted by injecting fluid through a port located beneath the skin. While food passes through the stomach normally, its passage is restricted by the smaller opening formed by the band. However, the Adjustable Gastric Band demonstrates less efficacy in managing type 2 diabetes and exerts only modest effects on metabolic health compared to alternative surgical interventions.

Biliopancreatic Diversion with Duodenal Switch

The Biliopancreatic Diversion with Duodenal Switch is a complex bariatric procedure that combines elements of sleeve gastrectomy and gastric bypass. Initially, a tube-shaped stomach pouch similar to that created in the sleeve gastrectomy is formed, reducing the stomach's capacity. Following this, a portion of the small intestine is rerouted to connect to the newly formed stomach pouch, diverting the food stream away from the majority of the small intestine.

This rerouting of the food stream bypasses approximately 75% of the small intestine, leading to a significant reduction in calorie and nutrient absorption. Consequently, patients typically need to supplement their diet with vitamins and minerals to prevent deficiencies. Moreover, the Biliopancreatic Diversion with Duodenal Switch influences intestinal hormones more profoundly than other bariatric procedures, resulting in reduced hunger, increased feelings of fullness, and improved blood sugar control. These metabolic effects make Biliopancreatic Diversion with Duodenal Switch particularly effective in treating type 2 diabetes, positioning it as one of the most potent approved metabolic surgeries available.

Single Anastomosis Duodenal-Ilea Bypass with Sleeve Gastrectomy

The Single Anastomosis Duodenal-Ilea Bypass with Sleeve Gastrectomy is similar to the Biliopancreatic Diversion with Duodenal Switch but with a simplified approach, the Single Anastomosis Duodeno-Ileal Bypass with Sleeve Gastrectomy involves only one surgical connection within the bowel, reducing surgical complexity and duration.

The surgical procedure commences similarly to a sleeve gastrectomy, creating a smaller tube-shaped stomach to restrict food intake. Following this, the first part of the small intestine is divided, and a loop of the intestine measured several feet from its end, is connected directly to the stomach. This single intestinal connection facilitates the passage of food from the pouch into the latter portion of the small intestine, where it mixes with digestive juices to enable adequate absorption of vitamins and minerals, ensuring nutritional balance. The Single Anastomosis Duodeno-Ileal Bypass with Sleeve Gastrectomy procedure not only promotes significant weight loss but also offers benefits such as reduced hunger, increased feelings of fullness, improved blood sugar control, and enhancement in diabetes management, making it a valuable option in the armamentarium of bariatric surgeries.

Who is a Candidate for Bariatric Surgery?

Bariatric surgery represents a critical intervention in the realm of weight management, typically considered a last resort for individuals who have grappled unsuccessfully with conventional weight loss methods. While diet, exercise, and lifestyle modifications are often the initial strategies recommended for weight loss, there exists a subset of individuals for whom these approaches prove ineffective or insufficient in addressing severe obesity and its associated health risks. Bariatric surgery emerges as a transformative option for these individuals, offering not only the prospect of significant weight loss but also the potential to alleviate or mitigate obesity-related comorbidities, such as type 2 diabetes, hypertension, and obstructive sleep apnea.

The success of bariatric surgery is contingent upon multiple factors, extending beyond the surgical procedure itself to encompass comprehensive post-operative care and adherence to lifestyle modifications. Following surgery, patients must commit to profound and enduring changes in their dietary habits, often transitioning to a regimen characterized by smaller portion sizes, emphasis on nutrient-dense foods, and avoidance of high-calorie, processed fare. Concurrently, a sustained commitment to regular physical activity is imperative, not only to optimize weight loss outcomes but also to promote cardiovascular health, musculoskeletal integrity, and overall well-being. In essence, bariatric surgery catalyzes profound lifestyle transformation, empowering individuals to adopt healthier habits that are instrumental in achieving and sustaining long-term weight loss success.

There is a clear eligibility criteria for individuals seeking bariatric surgery, with Body Mass Index serving as a foundational metric alongside the presence of obesity-related co-morbidities. A Body Mass Index exceeding 35, in conjunction with conditions such as diabetes, hypertension, or sleep apnea, signifies a heightened risk profile warranting consideration for surgical intervention. Moreover, individuals with a Body Mass Index surpassing 40, indicative of severe obesity, may derive substantial benefits from bariatric surgery, with the potential for profound improvements in both physical health and quality of life. Nevertheless, while these criteria provide a framework for candidacy assessment, decisions regarding bariatric surgery candidates are nuanced and multifaceted, informed by comprehensive evaluations of patients' medical histories, individual risk profiles, and psycho-social factors.

Despite the transformative potential of bariatric surgery, it is not devoid of challenges, risks, and limitations. Patients embarking on this journey must navigate a complex landscape of per-operative preparations, surgical procedures, and post-operative adjustments, guided by a multidisciplinary team of healthcare professionals. Furthermore, bariatric surgery necessitates a lifelong commitment to sustained behavioral change, encompassing dietary adherence, physical activity engagement, and ongoing medical follow-up. Moreover, there exist certain contraindications to bariatric surgery, including untreated psychiatric disorders, substance abuse issues, and plans for imminent pregnancy, underscoring the importance of comprehensive patient assessment and individualized care planning. Ultimately, the decision to pursue bariatric surgery represents a profound and deeply personal choice, requiring careful consideration, informed deliberation, and collaborative engagement with healthcare providers to optimize outcomes and enhance overall health and well-being.

3

Understanding Obesity

Definition of Obesity

Obesity is characterized by an excessive accumulation of fat, both globally and in specific regions of the body, leading to an increased risk of adverse health outcomes. Unlike acute illnesses, the definition of obesity does not necessitate the presence of obesity-related complications but rather signifies an elevated risk for their development. This broader perspective allows for the implementation of weight management strategies aimed at both treating existing conditions and preventing their onset. It is essential to recognize that thresholds for excess adiposity can vary based on individual factors such as body composition and fat distribution, highlighting the need for tailored approaches to weight assessment and intervention.

Ideally, an effective classification system for obesity would rely on a practical measurement accessible to healthcare providers across different settings, accurately predict health risks, and inform treatment strategies and goals. While precise measures of body fat, such as underwater weighing or imaging techniques like DEXA scanning and MRI, offer superior accuracy, they are impractical for routine clinical use. Estimates of body fat obtained through methods like Body Mass Index calculation and waist circumference measurement, while less precise, still offer valuable insights and are readily obtainable in various healthcare settings.

It is important to acknowledge two key considerations regarding current thresholds used to diagnose obesity. Firstly, the relationship between body weight or fat distribution and health conditions exists along a continuum, with increased risk extending beyond traditional Body Mass Index cutoffs. For instance, the risk of type 2 diabetes and premature mortality can be elevated even below the Body Mass Index threshold for obesity. Early intervention strategies aimed at preventing further weight gain or facilitating weight loss can yield significant health benefits in these earlier stages. Secondly, historical associations between rising Body Mass Index thresholds and the presence or severity of comorbidities may be evolving due to advancements in obesity-related treatments. For example, improved management of cardiovascular conditions has contributed to declines in atherosclerotic cardiovascular mortality rates, despite rising obesity rates. This underscores the importance of regularly updating epidemiological data on the health outcomes associated with overweight and obesity, considering factors such as healthcare utilization, medication usage, and treatment procedures in addition to morbidity and mortality statistics.

Causes and Contributing Factors

Dietary patterns and lifestyle choices exert profound influences on the development and progression of obesity and overweight conditions, shaping individuals' overall health trajectories. Among the most prevalent dietary factors contributing to these issues is the consumption of processed or fast food, which has become increasingly pervasive in modern society. These foods are often characterized by their high fat, sugar, and calorie content, offering little in terms of essential nutrients and fiber. Regular intake of processed or fast food not only contributes to excessive caloric intake but also undermines efforts to maintain a balanced diet, leading to weight gain and associated health complications over time.

In addition to dietary habits, alcohol consumption represents another significant lifestyle factor implicated in the obesity epidemic. Alcoholic beverages are energy-dense, containing a substantial number of calories per serving. Excessive alcohol consumption can contribute to weight gain by providing surplus energy that is stored as fat in the body. Moreover, alcohol consumption may also influence dietary behaviors, as it can impair judgment and increase appetite, leading individuals to consume larger portions or make less healthy food choices. Thus, moderating alcohol intake is crucial for individuals seeking to manage their weight effectively and improve their overall health outcomes.

Addressing the complex interplay between diet, lifestyle, and weight management requires a multifaceted approach that encompasses dietary modifications, increased physical activity, and behavioral changes. Strategies aimed at reducing the consumption of processed or fast food and moderating alcohol intake can serve as foundational components of effective weight management interventions. By fostering awareness of dietary patterns and promoting healthier lifestyle choices, individuals can take proactive steps towards achieving and maintaining a healthy weight, thereby mitigating the risk of obesity-related health complications and enhancing overall well-being.

Health Risks Associated with Obesity

Obesity represents far more than a mere cosmetic issue; it constitutes a significant medical problem with profound implications for overall health and well-being. Individuals affected by obesity face an elevated risk of developing a multitude of chronic diseases and health complications, underscoring the urgent need for effective prevention and management strategies. Among the myriad health conditions associated with obesity, cardiovascular diseases loom large, encompassing ailments such as heart disease, hypertension, and high cholesterol levels. These conditions can manifest as a result of the strain excess body weight places on the heart and blood vessels, increasing the likelihood of adverse cardiovascular events and complications.

Furthermore, obesity serves as a primary risk factor for the development of type 2 diabetes, a metabolic disorder characterized by impaired insulin function and elevated blood sugar levels. The intricate interplay between obesity and insulin resistance contributes to the pathogenesis of diabetes, heightening individuals' susceptibility to this debilitating condition. Additionally, obesity is closely linked to liver disease, including non-alcoholic fatty liver disease and nonalcoholic steatohepatitis, which can progress to more severe forms of liver damage and compromise overall liver function.

Moreover, obesity is intricately linked to the development of obstructive sleep apnea, a sleep disorder characterized by recurrent episodes of interrupted breathing during sleep. Excessive adipose tissue in the neck and throat region can obstruct the airway, leading to disruptions in breathing patterns and impaired sleep quality. Left untreated, sleep apnea can significantly impact daytime functioning and increase the risk of cardiovascular complications. Furthermore, obesity has been implicated in the pathogenesis of certain cancers, including breast, colorectal, and prostate cancer, highlighting the pervasive influence of excess body weight on diverse aspects of health and disease risk.

4

Evolution of Bariatric Surgery

Historical Perspective

The historical evolution of bariatric surgery traces back to ancient times, with accounts suggesting that the earliest form of such intervention occurred in 10th-century Spain. Legend has it that D. Sancho, King of Leon, sought treatment for his obesity from the renowned Jewish physician Hasdai Ibn Shaprut in Cordoba. The treatment involved suturing the king's lips and providing him with a liquid diet consisting of a concoction called teriaca, which included opium among its ingredients, inducing weight loss. This historical anecdote, albeit anecdotal, underscores the long-standing recognition of obesity as a medical concern warranting intervention, albeit primitive by modern standards.

The dawn of modern bariatric surgery can be attributed to pioneering efforts in the mid-20th century, marked by the introduction of the jejuno-ileal bypass. This procedure aimed to address severe dyslipidemia by rerouting the small intestine, albeit with considerable metabolic consequences and adverse effects. Subsequent refinements led to the development of the gastric bypass, which emerged as the first recognized bariatric surgery. The procedure underwent iterative enhancements, evolving from horizontal gastric transections to smaller pouches and improved reconstruction techniques, such as the Roux-en-Y loop, which minimized complications like bile reflux.

The advent of laparoscopic techniques heralded a new era in bariatric surgery, marked by increased safety, reduced invasiveness, and improved outcomes. Laparoscopic gastric bypasses revolutionized the field, paving the way for exponential growth in surgical interventions for obesity worldwide. Subsequent innovations, such as the Mini-Gastric Bypass and purely restrictive procedures like the gastric band, expanded the treatment armamentarium, offering tailored options for diverse patient populations. Despite the complexity and challenges inherent in these procedures, advancements in surgical techniques and increasing experience have propelled bariatric surgery into the forefront of obesity management, underscoring its pivotal role in addressing this burgeoning public health concern.

Advances in Surgical Techniques

The evolution of bariatric surgery has witnessed the integration of cutting-edge technologies, particularly robotics and laparoscopy, offering promising avenues for improved patient outcomes. In the context of gastric bypass procedures, both robotic and laparoscopic techniques have demonstrated comparable efficacy in terms of hospitalization duration, weight loss, weight regain, and 30-day mortality. However, robotic surgery has emerged as a favorable option, showcasing lower rates of bleeding, mortality, transfusions, and infections, thereby enhancing perioperative safety.

In the realm of revisional bariatric surgery, the robotic approach has showcased distinct advantages over laparoscopy, exhibiting fewer complications, shorter hospital stays, and reduced need for conversion to open surgery. Despite requiring more time in the operating room, the robotic platform has offered a more streamlined and efficient pathway for addressing complex cases, underscoring its utility in challenging surgical scenarios. Conversely, in sleeve gastrectomy procedures, robotic techniques have presented some trade-offs, necessitating more time and longer postoperative stays compared to laparoscopy. Nonetheless, they have demonstrated lower rates of transfusions and bleeding, highlighting their potential for minimizing intraoperative risks.

However, it's essential to acknowledge that while robotic surgeries hold promise for enhancing surgical precision and reducing complications, they also entail higher costs and potential complexities in postoperative management. The review also delves into the emerging single-anastomosis duodeno-ileal switch, revealing comparable outcomes between robotic and laparoscopic approaches, albeit with slightly longer operative times for robotic procedures. Overall, robotic technology in bariatric surgery represents a safe and effective modality, offering incremental benefits in select cases, albeit with nuanced considerations regarding operative time and resource utilization.

Future Direction

Despite the numerous advantages offered by bariatric surgery, some patients are hesitant to undergo current operative procedures due to concerns about potential complications, the necessity for adjustments involving needle punctures, or a desire to avoid alterations to their anatomy. This has led to a notable unmet need in the field, prompting exploration and development of innovative approaches. Among these are gastrointestinal neuromodulation techniques, including stimulating or blocking nervous pathways using electrical pulse generators, sleeve gastrectomy, intragastric balloons, intraluminal sleeves, and various other endoscopic procedures.

An example of neuromodulation is implantable gastric stimulation, where bipolar leads are laparoscopically implanted into the seromuscular layer of the stomach wall along the lesser curvature. These leads are then connected to an electrical pulse generator positioned subcutaneously along the abdominal wall. While the precise mechanism through which gastric stimulation induces weight loss is still being investigated, potential mechanisms include fundic expansion, vagal nerve stimulation, reduction in gastric emptying, and alterations in gut hormone activity. Despite variability in weight loss outcomes further research is needed to refine this technology despite its proven safety record.

Sleeve gastrectomy represents another evolving option for weight loss, serving either as a primary procedure or as the initial stage in a staged approach for exceptionally large patients or those deemed high-risk. During this operation, the greater curvature of the stomach is excised, leaving behind a tubular section along the lesser curvature. While the precise mechanism underlying weight loss remains unclear, it is believed to involve a reduction in calorie intake and appetite due to gastric restriction. Concerns exist regarding the potential long-term dilation of the remaining narrow stomach tube, necessitating further data collection for it to be considered a mainstream bariatric procedure.

Natural orifice transluminal endoscopic surgery represents a burgeoning concept in minimally invasive surgery, with applications being explored in bariatric procedures. Researchers are developing instruments and techniques aimed at limiting oral intake or mimicking the effects of gastric bypass. These include the implantation of intragastric balloons, intestinal sleeves, and methods for gastric partitioning and gastrojejunostomy. However, the efficacy, durability, and safety of these novel procedures require extensive validation before widespread adoption can be considered.

5

Preparing for Surgery

Preoperative Evaluation
The preoperative evaluation for bariatric surgery encompasses a meticulous and multifaceted process designed to provide a thorough understanding of the patient's health status, medical history, and psychological readiness for the impending surgical intervention. By thoroughly evaluating the patient's health status before surgery, healthcare providers can optimize baseline health and minimize surgical risks, ultimately leading to improved outcomes, including enhanced weight loss success.

One of the primary goals of the preoperative assessment is to identify and address any underlying medical conditions that could pose challenges during the surgical procedure or affect recovery afterward. A thorough review of the patient's medical history is conducted to identify any preexisting conditions that may impact surgery or recovery. This includes an in-depth exploration of past medical conditions, surgical procedures, medication history, allergies, and familial predispositions to obesity-related disorders. For example, conditions such as cardiovascular disease, diabetes, hypertension, and respiratory disorders may increase the risk of complications during anesthesia and surgery. By identifying these conditions early on, healthcare providers can implement appropriate management strategies to optimize the patient's health status before proceeding with surgery.

In addition to identifying medical conditions, the preoperative assessment also allows healthcare providers to evaluate the patient's overall fitness for surgery. This may involve assessing factors such as nutritional status, functional capacity, and any lifestyle habits that could impact surgical outcomes. For instance, patients who are malnourished or have poor nutritional status may be at increased risk of complications during surgery and may benefit from nutritional supplementation or dietary interventions before the procedure.

Furthermore, the preoperative assessment provides an opportunity for healthcare providers to educate patients about the importance of lifestyle modifications both before and after surgery. This may include counseling on dietary changes, exercise programs, smoking cessation, and alcohol consumption, all of which can play a significant role in optimizing surgical outcomes and promoting long-term weight loss success.

Physical examination is paramount in assessing the extent of obesity and its impact on overall health. Vital signs, body mass index, and waist circumference are meticulously assessed. Additionally, physical manifestations of obesity, such as skin changes, joint issues, and respiratory abnormalities, are carefully examined to gauge severity and anticipate surgical challenges.

Psychological evaluation is integral to ensuring the patient's emotional readiness for surgery. Mental health professionals conduct structured interviews and assessments to evaluate factors such as motivation, coping mechanisms, and understanding of the surgical procedure. Screening for psychiatric disorders, eating disorders, and substance abuse helps identify psychological barriers that may affect postoperative adherence.

Laboratory investigations provide objective data on metabolic parameters, organ function, and nutritional status. Blood tests assess glucose levels, lipid profile, liver function, renal function, and nutritional markers such as vitamin levels. These tests offer valuable insights into overall health and help identify any underlying issues requiring attention before surgery.

Furthermore, additional assessments may be performed based on individual patient needs. This may include specialized imaging studies, such as echocardiography or pulmonary function tests, to assess cardiovascular or respiratory function. Consultations with other medical specialists, such as cardiologists or pulmonologists, may also be sought to address specific concerns.

Overall, the preoperative evaluation for bariatric surgery is a comprehensive and collaborative effort involving multiple disciplines. By thoroughly assessing physical, psychological, and metabolic health, healthcare providers can identify potential risks, tailor the surgical approach, and provide appropriate support to ensure successful outcomes in the patient's weight loss journey.

Diet and Lifestyle Changes

Diet and lifestyle changes are integral components of the bariatric surgery journey, playing a crucial role in maximizing the effectiveness of the procedure and supporting long-term weight loss success. Before undergoing bariatric surgery, patients are typically advised to make significant adjustments to their diet and lifestyle habits to prepare for the procedure and optimize outcomes.

One of the primary goals of preoperative dietary modifications is to help patients achieve a healthier weight and reduce the size of the liver before surgery. This often involves following a low-calorie, high-protein diet to facilitate weight loss and shrink the liver, which can make the surgical procedure safer and more technically feasible. Additionally, reducing the intake of high-calorie and high-fat foods can help improve metabolic parameters and prepare the body for the changes that will occur after surgery.

Following bariatric surgery, particularly during the initial stages of recovery and weight loss, it's crucial to adhere to a carefully planned dietary regimen to support healing, promote weight loss, and ensure optimal nutritional intake. One key aspect of this regimen is controlling caloric intake, with recommended daily limits typically ranging from 500 to 700 calories during the first 12 months post-surgery. However, it's essential to avoid exceeding 1,000 calories per day to prevent overeating and potential complications.

A well-designed bariatric diet focuses on maximizing protein intake while minimizing consumption of carbohydrates and sugars. Protein plays a vital role in supporting muscle health, promoting satiety, and aiding in the healing process following surgery. Therefore, it's recommended to prioritize protein-rich foods such as lean meats, poultry, fish, eggs, dairy products, and plant-based protein sources like legumes and tofu. These foods should be included in each meal and snack to ensure adequate protein intake throughout the day.

In addition to protein, vegetables are another important component of the post-bariatric diet. Vegetables are nutrient-dense, low in calories, and high in fiber, vitamins, and minerals, making them an ideal choice for supporting overall health and wellness. Incorporating a variety of colorful vegetables into meals can help provide essential nutrients while promoting feelings of fullness and satisfaction. Non-starchy vegetables such as leafy greens, broccoli, cauliflower, bell peppers, and carrots are particularly beneficial choices.

While protein and vegetables should form the foundation of the bariatric diet, it's essential to limit the intake of carbohydrates and sugars, which can contribute to weight regain and metabolic issues. Foods high in refined carbohydrates and added sugars, such as sugary snacks, candies, baked goods, and processed foods, should be minimized or avoided altogether. Instead, focus on consuming complex carbohydrates from sources like whole grains, fruits, and legumes, which provide sustained energy and essential nutrients without causing rapid spikes in blood sugar levels.

Overall, following a well-designed dietary regimen that emphasizes high protein and vegetable intake while limiting carbohydrates and sugars is essential for achieving successful weight loss and maintaining long-term health after bariatric surgery. Working closely with a registered dietitian or nutritionist can help ensure that dietary needs are met, nutritional deficiencies are prevented, and dietary goals are achieved safely and effectively.

In addition to dietary changes, lifestyle modifications such as increasing physical activity and adopting healthier habits are essential components of preoperative preparation. Regular exercise not only aids in weight loss but also helps improve cardiovascular health, increase muscle mass, and enhance overall fitness levels. Patients are encouraged to engage in regular physical activity, such as walking, swimming, or cycling, to strengthen their bodies and improve their overall health before surgery.

Furthermore, preoperative counseling and education are essential components of the bariatric surgery process, helping patients understand the importance of dietary and lifestyle changes both before and after surgery. Patients are typically provided with guidance on portion control, meal planning, nutrient intake, and behavior modification techniques to support long-term success. Counseling sessions may also address emotional eating, stress management, and coping strategies to help patients develop healthier relationships with food and make sustainable lifestyle changes.

Following surgery, patients undergo a gradual transition to a modified diet that consists of small, frequent meals that are high in protein and low in carbohydrates and fats. This postoperative diet is designed to promote healing, prevent complications, and facilitate weight loss while providing essential nutrients to support recovery. Over time, patients are gradually able to reintroduce more varied foods into their diet, although portion control and mindful eating remain essential principles for long-term success.

In summary, diet and lifestyle changes are fundamental aspects of the bariatric surgery process, both before and after the procedure. By making significant adjustments to their diet and habits, patients can optimize their health, improve surgical outcomes, and achieve long-lasting weight loss success. Comprehensive support from healthcare providers, including nutrition counseling, exercise guidance, and behavioral therapy, is essential to help patients navigate these changes and adopt healthier lifestyles for life.

Psychological Preparation and Financial Consideration

Psychological preparation and financial considerations are vital aspects of the bariatric surgery journey, significantly impacting the overall success and satisfaction of patients undergoing this transformative procedure.

Psychological preparation involves comprehensive evaluation and counseling to ensure that patients are mentally and emotionally prepared for the challenges and changes associated with bariatric surgery. This process typically includes an assessment of the patient's mental health history, current psychological functioning, motivation, expectations, and readiness for lifestyle modifications. Psychologists or mental health professionals evaluate factors such as emotional eating, body image concerns, coping strategies, and support systems to identify any potential barriers to success and develop tailored interventions to address them.

Patients undergoing bariatric surgery may experience a range of emotions, including excitement, anxiety, fear, and uncertainty, both before and after the procedure. Psychological preparation aims to equip patients with the tools and strategies they need to navigate these emotional ups and downs effectively. This may involve providing education about the psychological aspects of obesity and weight loss, teaching stress management techniques, promoting self-awareness and self-compassion, and offering support and encouragement throughout the journey.

Setting realistic expectations is essential for success on the bariatric surgery journey. Rather than envisioning an idealized version of yourself, it's important to recognize that significant weight loss will require dedication, patience, and adherence to a structured meal plan.

A realistic approach involves understanding that weight loss will occur gradually over time, rather than overnight. By following a carefully crafted meal plan and incorporating healthy lifestyle changes, you can expect to see noticeable improvements in your weight and overall health within about six months.

It's crucial to remember that bariatric surgery is not a quick fix, but rather a tool to support long-term weight loss and improved well-being. While the initial months following surgery may bring significant changes, sustained success requires an ongoing commitment to dietary guidelines, regular exercise, and behavioral modifications.

By maintaining realistic expectations and staying dedicated to your post-surgery regimen, you can achieve meaningful and sustainable results on your bariatric journey. With the support of your healthcare team and loved ones, you'll be better equipped to navigate the challenges and celebrate the successes along the way.

Financial considerations are another important aspect of the bariatric surgery process, as the procedure can be costly and may not always be covered by insurance. Patients need to explore their insurance coverage options and understand the financial implications of bariatric surgery, including out-of-pocket expenses, co-payments, deductibles, and any coverage limitations or exclusions. Some insurance plans may require authorization or documentation of medical necessity before approving coverage for bariatric surgery, and patients may need to meet specific criteria or undergo certain evaluations or tests to qualify for coverage.

For patients without insurance coverage or facing significant out-of-pocket expenses, financial assistance options may be available, such as payment plans, medical loans, or financing programs offered by healthcare providers or third-party organizations. Patients should also consider the long-term costs associated with bariatric surgery, including follow-up care, nutritional supplements, and potential complications or revisions, and budget accordingly.

Psychological preparation and financial considerations are essential components of the bariatric surgery process, ensuring that patients are mentally and emotionally prepared for the procedure and equipped to manage the associated challenges and changes effectively. By addressing psychological factors and understanding the financial implications of bariatric surgery, patients can maximize their chances of success and achieve long-term weight loss and improved health outcomes. Comprehensive support from healthcare providers, including psychological counseling and financial counseling, is essential to help patients navigate these aspects of the bariatric surgery journey successfully.

6

The Surgical Process

Overview of the Surgery

Metabolic and bariatric surgeries stand as the culmination of decades of relentless refinement and innovation within the realm of medical science. These procedures represent some of the most thoroughly scrutinized treatments in modern medicine, characterized by their evolution towards utilizing minimally invasive surgical techniques, such as laparoscopic and robotic surgery. The embrace of these advanced methods has ushered in a new era marked by a host of benefits for patients, including diminished pain, reduced incidence of complications, shorter hospitalization periods, and expedited recovery times. Indeed, the safety profile of metabolic and bariatric operations often surpasses that of more traditional surgeries, such as gallbladder removal, hysterectomy, and hip replacement, positioning them as pillars of contemporary medical care.

At their core, metabolic and bariatric surgeries are designed to effect transformative changes within the anatomy of the stomach and intestines, thereby addressing the complex and multifaceted challenge of obesity and its associated comorbidities. These procedures typically entail interventions aimed at reducing the size of the stomach and modifying the gastrointestinal tract's architecture, often through methods like rerouting or bypassing sections of the intestine. By implementing these alterations, these surgeries exert a profound impact on both food intake and nutrient absorption, leading to a re-calibration of hunger signals and an enhancement of satiety sensations. Consequently, individuals undergoing these procedures find themselves better equipped to achieve and sustain a healthy weight, thereby ushering in significant improvements in overall metabolic health.

On the day of surgery, patients are admitted to the hospital or surgical facility, where they undergo the chosen bariatric procedure under the care of skilled medical professionals and the influence of general anesthesia. The specific surgical approach employed is tailored to the individual's unique circumstances, with considerations such as the type of operation selected (e.g., gastric bypass, sleeve gastrectomy, or gastric banding) guiding the surgeon's decisions. Throughout the procedure, which typically involves making small incisions in the abdomen, specialized instruments are utilized to execute precise modifications to the digestive system, facilitating weight loss and initiating metabolic transformations.

Following the completion of the surgical intervention, patients receive attentive postoperative care and monitoring in dedicated recovery areas before being transitioned to hospital rooms or designated recovery spaces. During this critical phase of recuperation, emphasis is placed on pain management, hydration, and mobilization, all of which play pivotal roles in fostering patient comfort and expediting the healing process.

As patients progress through the postoperative period, they are gradually guided in transitioning from a liquid diet to solid foods, a process overseen and facilitated by their healthcare providers.

While all surgical procedures inherently carry risks, bariatric surgeries performed at accredited centers consistently uphold stringent safety standards and boast commendable low complication rates. The attainment of successful outcomes hinges on the collaborative efforts of a multidisciplinary team of healthcare professionals, comprising surgeons, dietitians, psychologists, nurse case managers, and obesity medicine specialists. Equally crucial is the active engagement of patients themselves, who are encouraged to embrace healthy lifestyle habits, adhere to recommended dietary guidelines, participate in regular physical activity, and faithfully adhere to prescribed vitamin and mineral supplementation protocols.

In essence, bariatric surgery represents not merely a single, isolated event but rather the initiation of a transformative journey toward lasting health and well-being. Patients benefit from ongoing support and guidance from their dedicated bariatric care teams, who remain steadfast in their commitment to providing comprehensive care and facilitating sustained success. Through a steadfast dedication to lifelong health and wellness, individuals embarking on the bariatric surgery journey can anticipate not only significant weight loss but also a remarkable enhancement in overall quality of life and vitality.

Hospital Stay and Recovery

Hospital stay and postoperative recovery following bariatric surgery are pivotal stages in the treatment trajectory, characterized by meticulous oversight, symptom management, and the implementation of multifaceted strategies aimed at fostering healing and acclimatization to surgical alterations. The duration of hospitalization after bariatric surgery is subject to considerable variance contingent upon diverse factors, encompassing the specific procedural modality undertaken, the patient's overarching health status, and the manifestation of any postoperative complications. While offering a foundational framework, it's imperative to acknowledge the inherent variability in individual experiences.

In the aftermath of bariatric surgery, patients typically undergo a brief hospitalization, spanning one to three days, although this temporal framework remains contingent upon the procedural intricacies and individualized patient parameters. Throughout this hospital sojourn, patients benefit from vigilant oversight by a cadre of healthcare professionals, including nurses, physicians, and ancillary support staff, who meticulously monitor vital signs, address pain management requisites, and promptly attend to emergent postoperative exigencies or complications.

Central to the postoperative convalescence paradigm is the meticulous management of pain, entailing a repertoire of interventions aimed at assuaging discomfort and fostering patient comfort. Such modalities span the spectrum from pharmacological interventions encompassing both intravenous and oral analgesics to non-pharmacological measures such as the judicious application of ice packs, strategic positioning aids, and relaxation techniques.

In tandem with pain mitigation endeavors, ensuring optimal hydration constitutes a salient prerogative during the nascent postoperative phase. Patients are exhorted to ingest clear liquids comprising water, broth, and sugar-free beverages to forestall dehydration and engender an expedited convalescence trajectory. Intravenous fluid administration may be judiciously employed as indicated to safeguard hydration equilibrium and preserve electrolyte homeostasis.

Promoting mobility and fostering early ambulation emerge as pivotal imperatives in orchestrating postoperative rehabilitation initiatives, and pivotal in averting sequelae such as venous thromboembolism and pulmonary compromise. Patients are encouraged to partake in gradual mobilization and ambulatory activities post-surgery, under the judicious supervision of healthcare personnel. Such initiatives serve to bolster circulatory perfusion, enhance pulmonary dynamics, and fortify overall physiological well-being.

The postoperative dietary continuum unfolds in a meticulously calibrated manner, with patients embarking on a progressive trajectory from clear liquid nourishment to denser liquids, pureed comestibles, and eventually solid sustenance over an extended temporal arc. This gradual dietary reconstitution facilitates the gastrointestinal tract's adaptation to surgical perturbations and mitigates the risk of complications such as emesis, dumping syndrome, and micronutrient deficiencies.

Amidst the hospitalization and subsequent convalescence phase, patients receive a wealth of education and support from a multidisciplinary assemblage of healthcare professionals, including surgeons, nursing personnel, dietitians, and psychological counselors. This collaborative cohort endeavors to furnish comprehensive guidance on postoperative care paradigms, dietary strictures, recommendations for physical activity integration, and adept strategies for negotiating lifestyle modifications.

Upon hospital discharge, patients transition into the home

convalescent milieu, where they dutifully adhere to prescribed dietary regimens, and activity directives, and diligently attend scheduled follow-up appointments with their healthcare custodians. The temporal arc of postoperative recovery is contingent upon the patient's individualized progress trajectory and the procedural modality undertaken, albeit most patients can anticipate a resumption of customary activities and occupational obligations within several weeks to a month post-surgery.

Hospitalization and postoperative convalescence epitomize seminal junctures in the bariatric surgery odyssey, wherein patients are shepherded through a continuum of comprehensive care and support aimed at fostering convalescence, curbing complications, and ushering in enduring success in their weight loss and health amelioration aspirations. By actively engaging in their rehabilitation journey and assiduously heeding the directives of their healthcare stewards, patients stand poised to harness the transformative potential of bariatric surgery, thereby auguring a future characterized by an enhanced quality of life and sustained well-being.

Postoperative Care

Postoperative care following bariatric surgery is a critical phase of the treatment journey, encompassing a comprehensive array of interventions aimed at promoting healing, managing symptoms, and facilitating the patient's transition to a new dietary and lifestyle regimen. This period, spanning from the immediate postoperative phase to long-term follow-up, plays a pivotal role in optimizing surgical outcomes, preventing complications, and supporting the patient's long-term success in achieving weight loss and improved health.

In the immediate postoperative period, patients are closely

monitored in the recovery area or intensive care unit to ensure their stability and safety following surgery. Vital signs, including heart rate, blood pressure, respiratory rate, and oxygen saturation, are monitored regularly to detect any signs of complications such as bleeding, infection, or respiratory distress. Pain management is initiated promptly to alleviate discomfort and promote patient comfort, typically through a combination of oral or intravenous analgesic medications.

After undergoing bariatric surgery, maintaining your health and well-being requires a multifaceted approach that encompasses various aspects of self-care and adherence to prescribed guidelines. One crucial aspect of postoperative care is ensuring adequate nutrient intake by taking vitamins and supplements regularly. Since bariatric surgery can affect the body's ability to absorb certain nutrients, supplementation is essential to prevent deficiencies and support overall health.

In addition to supplementation, focusing on ingesting high-quality nutrients through your diet is paramount. Emphasizing lean proteins, fruits, vegetables, and whole grains can help ensure that you're meeting your body's nutritional needs while promoting healing and supporting weight loss efforts. Working with a registered dietitian or nutritionist can be invaluable in developing a balanced and nutritious eating plan tailored to your individual needs and preferences.

Hydration is another essential aspect of postoperative care, as patients may be at risk of dehydration due to restricted oral intake and potential fluid losses during surgery. Intravenous fluids may be administered as needed to maintain hydration and electrolyte balance until the patient can tolerate oral fluids adequately. Encouraging early ambulation and mobility is also crucial for preventing complications such as blood clots and promoting circulation, lung function, and overall recovery.

Dietary progression is carefully managed during the postoperative period, with patients initially starting on a clear liquid diet and gradually advancing to thicker liquids, pureed foods, and eventually solid foods over several weeks. Patients receive guidance from dietitians and nutritionists on appropriate portion sizes, macronutrient balance, and strategies for adapting to the dietary restrictions and requirements imposed by bariatric surgery. Nutritional supplements, including vitamins and minerals, may be prescribed to prevent deficiencies and support overall health and healing.

In addition to physical recovery, patients undergo psychological and emotional adjustment following bariatric surgery, as they adapt to changes in body image, eating habits, and lifestyle. Psycho-social support is provided through counseling, support groups, and educational resources to help patients navigate these transitions, address any emotional challenges or concerns, and develop coping strategies for managing stress, cravings, and behavioral changes. Participating in support groups or counseling sessions can provide invaluable emotional and psychological support as you navigate the challenges and changes associated with bariatric surgery. Connecting with others who have undergone similar experiences can offer encouragement, inspiration, and practical tips for success. Additionally, individual or group therapy sessions can help you address any emotional issues, body image concerns, or behavioral patterns that may arise during your weight loss journey.

Long-term follow-up care is an integral component of postoperative management, ensuring ongoing support, monitoring, and optimization of outcomes in the months and years following surgery. Patients attend regular follow-up appointments with their surgical team, including surgeons, dietitians, psychologists, and other healthcare professionals, to assess progress, address any issues or concerns, and provide ongoing guidance and support for maintaining weight loss, adhering to dietary and lifestyle recommendations, and managing any potential complications or comorbidities.

Physical activity is another crucial component of postoperative care, contributing to weight loss, muscle strength, cardiovascular health, and overall well-being. Engaging in regular exercise, such as walking, swimming, cycling, or strength training, can help you maintain your weight loss, increase your energy levels, and improve your mood. Start slowly and gradually increase the intensity and duration of your workouts as you build strength and endurance.

Ultimately, your dedication to this multifaceted plan is crucial for ensuring both your emotional and physical well-being after bariatric surgery. By prioritizing nutrient intake, attending follow-up appointments, engaging in regular exercise, and seeking support when needed, you can maximize the benefits of surgery and achieve long-term success in your weight loss and health improvement goals. Also, adherence to the prescribed dietary phases is crucial for promoting successful outcomes and ensuring a smooth transition to solid foods following bariatric surgery. Patients should closely follow the guidance of their healthcare providers and dietitians, attend regular follow-up appointments, and make adjustments to their diet as needed to support their weight loss and overall health goals. By following the recommended dietary progression and adopting healthy eating habits, patients can maximize the benefits of bariatric surgery and achieve long-term success in their weight loss journey. Overall, postoperative care following bariatric surgery is a multifaceted and dynamic process that requires a coordinated and multidisciplinary approach to address the physical, psychological, and nutritional needs of patients throughout their recovery and beyond. By providing comprehensive support, education, and guidance, healthcare providers can empower patients to achieve successful outcomes and sustain long-term improvements in their health and quality of life.

7

Life After Bariatric Surgery

Dietary Guidelines and Nutrition

After undergoing bariatric surgery, patients typically progress through several phases of dietary adaptation, each carefully designed to support healing, promote weight loss, and minimize discomfort. These phases gradually introduce different textures and consistencies of food while ensuring adequate nutrient intake and promoting adherence to postoperative guidelines. Below is an overview of the various phases of the post-bariatric surgery diet plan:

Phase 1: Clear Liquid Diet (Weeks 1 and 2)

During the initial postoperative period, patients are instructed to consume clear liquids only to allow the gastrointestinal tract to rest and heal. Clear liquids include water, broth, sugar-free gelatin, and clear fruit juices without pulp. These liquids provide hydration and essential electrolytes while minimizing strain on the digestive system. It's essential to sip liquids slowly and avoid carbonated beverages and caffeinated drinks during this phase.

Phase 2A: Full Liquid Diet (N/A)

In some bariatric programs, a full liquid diet phase may be included between the clear liquid and pureed diet phases. Full liquids are more substantial than clear liquids and include items such as milk, yogurt, protein shakes, and cream-based soups. This phase provides additional protein and calories while still maintaining a liquid or semi-liquid consistency. However, not all programs include this phase, and some patients may progress directly to the pureed diet phase.

Phase 2B: Pureed Diet (Weeks 3 and 4)

The pureed diet phase introduces foods with a smooth, blended consistency to facilitate easier digestion and reduce the risk of discomfort or irritation. Pureed foods may include strained soups, cottage cheese, yogurt, mashed vegetables, and soft fruits. It's essential to avoid foods with chunks or solid pieces during this phase and focus on consuming small, frequent meals to prevent overeating and promote satiety. Additionally, incorporating protein supplements into the diet helps ensure adequate protein intake during this early stage of recovery.

Phase 3: Adaptive/Soft Diet (Months 2 and 3)

As the digestive system continues to heal and adapt, patients progress to the adaptive or soft diet phase, which allows for the gradual introduction of more solid foods with softer textures. Foods in this phase may include cooked vegetables, tender meats, fish, eggs, tofu, and well-cooked grains. It's essential to chew food thoroughly and eat slowly to aid digestion and prevent discomfort. Patients should also continue to prioritize protein intake and stay hydrated by consuming plenty of fluids throughout the day.

Exercise and Physical Activity

Bariatric surgery is an effective intervention for significant weight loss and the improvement of obesity-related conditions. However, achieving a healthier lifestyle extends beyond the surgery itself. Incorporating regular exercise into the post-operative care plan is crucial for sustaining weight loss and enhancing overall well-being. Studies consistently demonstrate that patients who engage in regular physical activity after bariatric surgery achieve greater weight loss at 12 and 24 months postoperative compared to those who do not exercise. Physical activity raises the number of calories burned, contributing to a greater caloric deficit and enhanced weight loss. Exercise, especially resistance training, helps maintain muscle mass during weight loss, which is essential for sustaining metabolic rate. Regular exercise boosts insulin sensitivity and cardiovascular health, lowering the risk of conditions such as type 2 diabetes and heart disease. A well-rounded exercise program for bariatric surgery patients should encompass aerobic activities, strength training, and flexibility exercises. Activities like walking, cycling, and swimming improve cardiovascular health and promote weight loss. Patients should start with low-impact exercises and gradually increase intensity. Engaging in resistance exercises 2-3 times a week helps build and preserve muscle mass, crucial for a healthy metabolism. Practices like yoga, stretching, and balance exercises enhance overall physical function and minimize injury risk.

Patients should consult their healthcare providers before beginning any exercise regimen to ensure it aligns with their health status and fitness level. A phased, progressive approach is typically recommended:

• Initial Phase (0-3 months post-surgery): Focus on light

activities such as short walks, gentle stretching, and light movements to aid healing and prevent complications.

- Intermediate Phase (3-6 months post-surgery): Gradually increase the duration and intensity of aerobic exercises and introduce light resistance training. Aim for at least 150 minutes of moderate-intensity aerobic activity per week.
- Advanced Phase (6+ months post-surgery): Continue to build on aerobic and strength training activities, aiming for a balanced and varied exercise routine that includes all major muscle groups.

While short-term studies emphasize the benefits of exercise within the first two years post-bariatric surgery, the long-term effects are still being researched. Regular exercise helps prevent weight regain, a common challenge after bariatric surgery. Physical activity is linked to reduced symptoms of depression and anxiety, contributing to better overall mental well-being. Patients who maintain an active lifestyle report higher satisfaction with their physical health, mobility, and overall quality of life.

Exercise and physical activity are vital components of a successful postoperative plan for bariatric surgery patients. By promoting greater weight loss, preserving muscle mass, and improving metabolic health, regular physical activity enhances the benefits of bariatric surgery and supports long-term health and well-being. Patients should collaborate with their healthcare teams to develop and maintain a personalized exercise regimen that evolves with their recovery and fitness levels. Commitment to an active lifestyle enables bariatric surgery patients to achieve lasting weight loss and an improved quality of life.

Managing Emotional and Psychological Changes

Bariatric surgery offers transformative benefits for those struggling with weight issues, leading to significant weight loss and an enhanced quality of life. However, alongside these physical changes, many patients experience emotional and psychological shifts, commonly referred to as mood changes after bariatric surgery. In this article, our experts will explore these emotional changes and provide advice on how to manage them effectively. It is common for patients to report mood swings following bariatric procedures. These emotional changes can range from feelings of euphoria and excitement to bouts of sadness and irritability. While these shifts may seem alarming, they are a normal part of the post-surgery experience.

Several factors can contribute to mood swings after gastric sleeve or other bariatric procedures, including:

- Hormonal Changes: Rapid weight loss can affect hormones like ghrelin and leptin, which play roles in mood regulation and appetite control.
- Nutritional Deficiencies: Post-surgery dietary restrictions can lead to nutritional deficiencies, impacting emotional well-being.
- Body Image and Self-Esteem: As the body undergoes dramatic changes, shifts in self-esteem and body image perception are common.
- Psychological Stress: Adapting to a new lifestyle and managing the expectations of successful weight loss can be emotionally challenging.

Patients experiencing mood changes after bariatric surgery can take several steps to manage their emotions effectively:

- Seek Support: Connect with a support group, therapist, or counselor specializing in post-bariatric emotional changes. Talking about your feelings can be incredibly helpful.
- Maintain Follow-Up Care: Regular follow-up appointments with your bariatric team are crucial for monitoring both physical and emotional well-being.
- Balanced Diet and Supplements: Ensure you are following your nutritional guidelines and taking prescribed supplements to address potential deficiencies.
- Stay Active: Regular physical activity can help improve mood and reduce stress.
- Set Realistic Expectations: Understand that bariatric surgery is a tool, not a magic solution, and that weight loss may not resolve all emotional challenges.

Understanding and managing the causes of mood swings after bariatric surgery is essential for a successful post-operative journey. By seeking support, maintaining follow-up care, ensuring nutritional balance, staying active, and setting realistic expectations, patients can effectively navigate these emotional changes and enjoy the full benefits of their transformative surgery.

8

Managing Complications and Side Effects

Early and Late Postoperative Complications
Postoperative complications following bariatric surgery can occur early or late. Acute care surgeons must be aware of common issues and management strategies due to the permanent anatomical changes from these procedures.

Anastomotic leaks are critical complications with high morbidity and mortality. Symptoms include persistent tachycardia, dyspnea, fever, and abdominal pain. Leaks are more likely in patients who have undergone revisional procedures or have a high Body Mass Index. Treatment may involve image-guided drainage or endoluminal interventions.

Stenosis is another significant concern. It is managed with endoscopic balloon dilation, though multiple treatments may be necessary. Sleeve gastrectomies and Roux-en-Y gastric bypasses have different management approaches due to variations in endoluminal pressure.

Postoperative bleeding, though less common, requires

prompt intervention. Endoscopic evaluation is crucial, and surgical exploration may be needed for hemodynamic instability.

Venous thromboembolism is a risk, especially in high-risk patients. Screening with CT angiogram and systemic anticoagulation are standard treatments.

Intragastric balloon complications, though rare, can be severe, including perforation and migration. Early recognition and intervention are vital, using endoscopic techniques for deflation and removal, and surgical options if necessary.

Complications from laparoscopic adjustable gastric band surgery are common. These include band slippage and tubing breakage. More severe problems include band erosion, acute obstruction, ischemia, and megaesophagus or pseudoachalasia. About 25% of patients need reoperation due to complications or insufficient weight loss.

Band slippage occurs in about 8% of patients, causing symptoms like vomiting, a feeling of fullness relieved by vomiting, and abdominal pain. Severe cases can lead to obstruction, ischemia, and stomach wall dilation. Treatment involves emptying the band of fluid, which often resolves the issue. Persistent symptoms may require emergency surgery to remove the band.

Band erosion happens in 0.31% to 1.96% of patients. Symptoms include abdominal pain, loss of food restriction, melena, and infection of the band port. Diagnosis is done through X-rays, CT scans, or upper endoscopy. Treatment involves antibiotics and referral to a bariatric surgeon. Complete or near-complete erosions can be removed endoscopically, while partial erosions might need laparoscopic removal.

Megaesophagus or pseudoachalasia can occur, causing difficulty swallowing, regurgitation, and vomiting. Diagnosis is made through X-rays or ultrasound. Treatment involves emptying the band and planning for elective band removal.

Roux-en-Y gastric bypass can also lead to complications. Patients may develop gallstones more frequently due to changes in bile flow and hormonal shifts. Symptoms can be atypical, and treatment usually involves laparoscopic cholecystectomy. More complex cases might need advanced endoscopic or surgical techniques.

Marginal ulcers occur in less than 5% of patients and can cause epigastric pain, bleeding, and sometimes perforation. Treatment involves resuscitation, endoscopy, and surgery if bleeding persists.

Internal hernias occur in about 2.5% of patients and can be difficult to diagnose. Symptoms are often vague but may include abdominal pain and bowel obstruction. Diagnosis may require imaging, though CT scans can miss some cases. Treatment typically involves prompt surgical intervention to prevent serious complications like volvulus and bowel ischemia.

Complications from bariatric surgery require early diagnosis and appropriate treatment. Patients often need surgical con-sultation and intervention to manage these serious conditions effectively.

Dumping Syndrome and Other Gastrointestinal Issues

Dumping syndrome after gastric bypass surgery is when food moves directly from your stomach pouch into your small intestine without being digested. There are two types of dumping syndrome: early and late. Early dumping happens 10 to 30 minutes after a meal, while late dumping happens 1 to 3 hours after eating.

Early dumping syndrome occurs because a dense mass of food is dumped into your small intestine early in digestion. The intestines sense that this food mass is too concentrated and release gut hormones. Your body reacts by shifting fluid from your bloodstream into your intestine, causing it to become fuller and bloated. Diarrhea often occurs 30 to 60 minutes later. Substances released by your intestine can affect heart rate and blood pressure, causing lightheadedness or even fainting.

Late dumping syndrome happens due to a decrease in blood sugar levels (reactive hypoglycemia). This is low blood sugar caused 1 to 3 hours after a large surge of insulin. Eating a meal high in starches or sugars can trigger this. Insulin levels can increase to high levels and then lower your blood sugar too much.

Dumping syndrome occurs in approximately 20% to 50% of people who have had gastric surgery. The severity of symptoms depends on the extent of the surgery.

Most people have early dumping symptoms. Typical early dumping symptoms include bloating, sweating, abdominal cramps and pain, nausea, facial flushing, stomach growling or rumbling, an urge to lie down after eating, heart palpitations and fast heartbeat, dizziness or fainting, diarrhea, and feeling full after eating only a small amount of food.

About one in four people have late dumping symptoms, which occur 1 to 3 hours after a meal. Late dumping symptoms include heart palpitations, sweating, hunger, confusion, fatigue, aggression, tremors, and fainting.

Your healthcare team will likely diagnose dumping syndrome based on your symptoms and when they occur. Tell your provider which foods or liquids give you symptoms. You may also need a glucose tolerance test or hydrogen breath test to help diagnose you.

The main treatment for dumping syndrome is dietary changes. These include not drinking liquids until at least 30 minutes after a meal, dividing your daily calories into six small meals, lying down for 30 minutes after a meal to help control symptoms, choosing complex carbohydrates like whole grains, fruits, and vegetables, avoiding foods high in simple carbohydrates, adding more protein, fiber, and fat to your meals, and stopping dairy foods if they cause problems.

Another option to slow gastric emptying is making your food thicker. Your healthcare provider may advise adding 15 grams of guar gum or pectin to each meal, though many people don't tolerate these additions well.

If dietary changes don't help, your healthcare provider may prescribe slow-release medicines. These are rare and often not effective. In severe cases, your healthcare provider may suggest tube feeding or corrective surgery.

Dumping syndrome symptoms can be distressing, leading some people to severely limit their food intake, which can cause more problems and even lead to malnutrition. Because dumping syndrome can become serious, it's important to talk with your healthcare provider when you first have symptoms.

Strategies for Coping and Seeking Support

For many people, food becomes a way to cope and comfort themselves. After weight loss surgery, this ability is disrupted due to smaller portions and food intolerances. Developing alternative and healthy coping skills is essential after weight loss surgery.

Obesity has many contributing factors and is not solely due to poor eating habits or lack of exercise. After weight loss surgery, it is important to make healthy dietary choices. Ensure that eating is not driven by emotions or emotional eating.

The mental aspect of weight loss surgery should not be ignored. Developing healthy coping skills can help with the changes that occur. Some people may mourn the loss of foods that once provided comfort or a sense of belonging. Seeking help from a mental health care provider can be beneficial to work through these feelings. Do not hesitate to contact a mental health professional if needed.

Effective coping techniques can be practiced before weight loss surgery. Spending time in nature can energize the body and calm the mind. Sunlight increases Vitamin D levels, which can improve mood and well-being.

Exercise has both mental and physical benefits after weight loss surgery. The natural chemical release from exercise has a calming effect and promotes a sense of well-being. Additionally, exercise aids in weight loss and positive body changes, which can improve mental and emotional health.

Music can soothe or energize the soul. Listen to music, sing along, or dance to enjoy its benefits. Journaling before and after surgery can provide perspective and track progress. Documenting body measurements, pictures, and weights can show how far you have come.

Mindfulness involves using all five senses to experience life and food fully. Take your time and be present in all experiences. Ask yourself if you are enjoying the moment, if it meets your needs, and if it is healthy for you.

Support groups with peers who understand your experiences can be valuable. There are many face-to-face and online support groups available. Treat yourself by practicing self-care through activities that relax or energize you, like getting a massage, manicure, or taking a class.

Distractions like hobbies, new skills, reading, games, or bubble baths can help calm and soothe the mind. Talking to a close friend or trusted therapist provides an opportunity to share and unload challenges.

Changing habits and coping skills takes practice and patience. Focus on small steps, goals, and achievements. Give yourself credit for the progress you have made. Remember how far you have come and the positive lifestyle changes you have achieved. If you experience setbacks, do not be hard on yourself. Move forward and continue working towards your goals.

9

Reaching The Goal

Journey of Transformation

The journey toward reclaiming health and vitality stands as a testament to the resilience of the human spirit and the transformative power of perseverance. It initiates upon returning home from surgery, marking a pivotal juncture where the seeds of change are sown, and the path to a healthier, more fulfilling life is laid out before them.

In the initial days post-surgery, there's a delicate dance between movement and rest as the body acclimates to the alterations brought about by the procedure. Encouraged to gradually reintegrate physical activity into their routine, it's equally crucial for them to allow necessary time and space for recuperation. Each step forward becomes a testament to their unwavering determination and commitment to reclaiming their well-being.

Amidst the physical challenges, the steadfast support of loved ones serves as a beacon of strength, offering solace, encouragement, and unwavering support. Their presence serves as a constant reminder that they are not alone in this journey, and together, they can surmount any obstacle standing in their path.

As the weeks unfold, the transformative effects of the surgery begin to manifest in subtle yet profound ways. Changes in appetite and eating habits emerge, signaling a seismic shift in their relationship with food. No longer driven by the insatiable cravings of the past, they find themselves attuned to their body's signals, savoring each bite with mindful awareness. The journey toward a healthier lifestyle transcends mere weight loss, evolving into a deeper, more harmonious connection with the body, nourishing it with the care and respect it deserves.

With newfound mobility and vitality, the world beckons with boundless opportunities for exploration and adventure. From strolls through sun-kissed meadows to exhilarating hikes amidst towering peaks, each outing becomes a celebration of their newfound freedom and resilience. Cultural pursuits once relegated to the realm of distant dreams now take center stage in their life, as they revel in the joy of shared experiences and meaningful connections.

Looking towards the future, the horizon shimmers with promise and possibility. Thoughts of starting a family or pursuing long-held passions take root, fueled by a newfound sense of confidence and self-assurance. The journey toward reclaiming health is about more than shedding excess weight; it's about rediscovering the boundless potential dormant within them and charting a course toward a brighter, more vibrant future.

Amidst the tapestry of challenges and triumphs, they come to a profound realization — they have broken free from the shackles of obesity. No longer defined by the limitations of the past, they now stand as a beacon of hope and inspiration, a testament to the indomitable power of the human spirit to rise above adversity and embrace the fullness of life. With each passing day, they continue to forge ahead, unwavering in their commitment to living their best life and savoring every precious moment along the way.

Challenges and Triumphs

Bariatric surgery stands as a transformative option for individuals battling severe obesity. Yet, this journey is laden with both hurdles and victories, stretching across the pre-operative phase to post-surgical recovery and beyond.

- Pre-Surgery Challenges:

Before the operating theater, patients traverse a maze of obstacles, including rigorous medical evaluations. These assessments delve deep into their health, identifying potential complications and ensuring they comprehend the risks and rewards. This phase often amplifies psychological struggles, with anxiety, fear, and body image issues casting shadows over the decision to undergo surgery. Moreover, preparing for bariatric surgery necessitates substantial lifestyle adjustments. Patients must overhaul their dietary habits, embrace physical activity, and bid farewell to detrimental behaviors like smoking and excessive drinking. Yet, perhaps the most formidable barrier lies in navigating the labyrinthine insurance approval process. Insurers wield strict criteria, making securing coverage akin to scaling a mountain.

- Triumphs:

Despite these challenges, bariatric surgery heralds remarkable triumphs, beginning with an upsurge in health. The shedding of excess weight begets a cascade of improvements, with conditions like type 2 diabetes, hypertension, and sleep apnea often receding into the background. As the numbers on the scale dwindle, patients find themselves liberated to partake in activities once shunned due to their weight. Enhanced mobility, elevated energy levels, and a newfound zest for life become their companions. Furthermore, the psychological benefits are profound. Many report a lightening of the emotional burden, with reduced symptoms of depression and anxiety ushering in a sense of tranquility. The surgery fosters empowerment, as patients seize the reins of their health, embarking on a journey of self-discovery and resilience.

- Post-Surgery Challenges:

Yet, the path to transformation is riddled with potholes, even after surgery. Dietary restrictions loom large, demanding adherence to strict guidelines to facilitate healing and stave off complications. The transition from liquid to solid foods requires discipline and patience, testing the resolve of even the most determined. Physical recovery is another battleground, with pain, discomfort, and fatigue shadowing the postoperative days. Emotional turbulence simmers beneath the surface as well, as patients grapple with the shifting sands of their relationship with food and body image. Complications, though rare, cast a pall over the journey, reminding patients of the fragility of their newfound health.

- Triumphs:

Nevertheless, amidst the challenges, triumphs emerge like beacons of hope. Weight loss becomes not merely a number on the scale but a testament to perseverance and dedication. Health issues that once loomed large recede into the distance, replaced by vitality and vigor. Medications are shed like unwanted baggage, and the specter of complications fades into oblivion. With each milestone reached, self-esteem soars to new heights, permeating every facet of life. Empowerment becomes the cornerstone of existence, as patients revel in their newfound agency, forging ahead on a path paved with resilience and determination.

Bariatric surgery is more than a medical procedure; it is a journey of transformation, fraught with challenges yet crowned with triumphs. Through perseverance and resilience, individuals emerge from the crucible of obesity, reborn into a life brimming with health, vitality, and empowerment.

Maintaining Weight Loss and Preventing Weight Regain

If you've had bariatric surgery, congratulations on taking a significant step forward in living a healthier life. Now, you might be wondering how to go about keeping the weight off that you've lost.

While bariatric surgery is an invaluable tool for losing weight, it's important to remember that surgery alone isn't a permanent solution to obesity. Practicing good eating and exercise habits is key to staying at a healthy weight.

It's so important after surgery to eat healthy foods, follow the bariatric protocol for nutrition that you are given, and stay active, or the disease and its comorbidities may return. In the first year to 18 months after surgery, most patients are diligent about sticking to good diet and exercise habits. But as they start to tolerate a wider variety of foods, many begin to eat more and exercise less. Weight loss slows down or plateaus before beginning to creep up.

Weight regain after bariatric surgery is most often related to diet, but it can happen for a variety of reasons. For example, a fistula (abnormal opening) may develop after gastric bypass surgery that allows food to enter the bigger stomach. Or, the sleeve from a sleeve gastrectomy may get too stretched to sufficiently limit food intake.

While weight regain is common after bariatric surgery, it's not inevitable. Start by recognizing that obesity is a chronic condition that causes your body to gain weight, making it a lifelong challenge. A dedicated bariatric team is your ally in the fight to lose weight and improve your health. Understanding this can help you stay committed to the necessary lifestyle changes.

Don't be ashamed if you begin regaining weight. Reach out to your bariatric team to help you determine why this is happening. They are here to help you succeed. You may benefit from one of the approved weight-loss medications or some simple coaching and support. Your team can offer tailored advice and interventions to help you get back on track.

Schedule regular visits with your bariatric team. Consistent follow-ups are crucial for keeping your weight loss on track and maintaining accountability. These regular check-ins can help identify any issues early and provide support and adjustments to your plan as needed.

Follow your recommended diet and nutrition plan diligently. Adhering to the diet and nutrition plan provided by your bariatric team will help ensure you get adequate nutrients and maintain your muscle mass. The goal is to eat a regular diet in smaller amounts, focusing on nutrient-dense foods that support your overall health and weight maintenance.

Avoid snacking or grazing. Snacking or grazing can prevent you from feeling full and add extra calories that will sabotage your weight loss. Stick to planned meals and snacks to keep your hunger and satiety cues in check.

Seek support when needed. If you have trouble maintaining the lifestyle changes that have been recommended for you, seek a weight-loss support group. Chances are you'll find others who are struggling with the same issues. If you feel you would benefit from individualized support, your bariatric team can connect you with someone who has been in your shoes to mentor you. Support from others who understand your journey can be incredibly motivating and helpful.

If you regain weight, dig deep inside yourself to remember why you sought bariatric surgery in the first place. Then recommit yourself to the goals you set out to achieve. You can do this! Remember that weight-loss surgery is currently the most effective way to lose excess weight and has the highest rates of weight maintenance in the long term. Success in bariatric surgery is defined as retaining 50 percent of weight loss five years after a patient's initial procedure. Rarely do patients gain all their weight back.

Should weight regain occur, know that it's not about failure and that there are options available to address it. From tailored counseling and behavioral therapy programs to weight-loss medications and laparoscopic revision surgery, your bariatric team is here to get you back on the road to better health. By staying proactive and utilizing the resources and support available to you, you can successfully maintain your weight loss and enjoy the benefits of your healthier lifestyle.

10

Conclusion

I n concluding this comprehensive exploration of bariatric surgery, it's evident that embarking on this transformative journey requires a deep understanding and commitment to various aspects of the process. Bariatric surgery represents a significant medical intervention aimed at addressing obesity and its associated health risks, offering individuals a pathway to substantial weight loss and improved well-being.

Beginning with an understanding of what bariatric surgery entails, we delved into the different types of procedures available, ranging from gastric bypass to sleeve gastrectomy, each with its unique mechanisms and outcomes. By understanding the nuances of these procedures, individuals can make informed decisions in collaboration with their healthcare providers.

Moreover, we discussed the criteria for candidacy, recognizing that while bariatric surgery can be life-changing, it's not suitable for everyone. Factors such as Body Mass Index, obesity-related health conditions, and previous weight loss efforts play a crucial role in determining eligibility, underscoring the importance of thorough evaluation and patient-provider communication.

Understanding obesity itself is paramount, as it provides the context for why bariatric surgery is often necessary. From exploring the definition and classification of obesity to examining its multi-factorial causes and contributing factors, we gained insights into the complex nature of this chronic condition and its far-reaching implications for health and well-being.

We also highlighted the health risks associated with obesity, ranging from cardiovascular disease to type 2 diabetes, underscoring the urgent need for effective interventions. By addressing obesity through bariatric surgery, individuals can mitigate these risks and improve their overall health outcomes, thereby enhancing their quality of life.

The evolution of bariatric surgery was a key theme throughout our exploration, tracing its historical roots to the latest advances in surgical techniques and future directions. From the pioneering efforts of early surgeons to the development of minimally invasive procedures and innovative approaches, the field of bariatric surgery continues to evolve, offering new hope for individuals struggling with obesity.

Preparation for surgery involves a multifaceted approach, encompassing preoperative evaluations, dietary and lifestyle modifications, psychological preparation, and financial considerations. By adequately preparing patients for the surgical process and postoperative recovery, healthcare providers can optimize outcomes and ensure patient safety and satisfaction.

Life after bariatric surgery is a journey filled with both challenges and triumphs. By adhering to dietary guidelines, engaging in regular physical activity, and managing emotional and psychological changes, individuals can navigate this journey successfully. Additionally, being vigilant about potential complications and side effects, such as dumping syndrome and nutritional deficiencies, is essential for long-term success.

Ultimately, maintaining weight loss and preventing weight regain requires ongoing commitment and support. By embracing lifestyle changes, seeking support from healthcare professionals and peers, and celebrating achievements along the way, individuals can achieve their health goals and experience lasting transformation.

In conclusion, bariatric surgery represents not just a procedure but a profound opportunity for individuals to reclaim their health and well-being. Through education, preparation, and ongoing support, individuals can embark on this journey with confidence, knowing that they have the tools and resources to achieve lasting success and enjoy a healthier, more fulfilling life.

11

Resources

Biliopancreatic diversion with duodenal switch (BPD/DS) - Mayo Clinic. (2022, June 25). https://www.mayoclinic.org/tests-procedures/biliopancreatic-diversion-with-duodenal-switch/about/pac-20385180

Bariatric surgery - Mayo Clinic. (2023, October 18). https://www.mayoclinic.org/tests-procedures/bariatric-surgery/about/pac-20394258

Am I a candidate for weight loss surgery? | Cleveland Clinic. (n.d.). Cleveland Clinic. https://my.clevelandclinic.org/departments/bariatric/candidate#:~:text=To%20be%20eligible%20for%20bariatric,having%20a%20BMI%20of%2040).

Obesity - Symptoms and causes - Mayo Clinic. (2023, July 22). Mayo Clinic. https://www.mayoclinic.org/diseases-conditions/obesity/symptoms-causes/syc-20375742#:~:text=Obesity%20isn't%20just%20a,sleep%20apnea%20and%20%20certain%20cancers.

Moshiri, M., Osman, S., Robinson, T. J., Khandelwal,

S., Bhargava, P., & Rohrmann, C. A. (2013). Evolution of Bariatric Surgery: a historical perspective. *American Journal of Roentgenology, 201*(1), W40–W48. https://doi.org/10.2214/ajr.12.10131

Faria, G. R. (2017, March 6). *A brief history of bariatric surgery.* https://www.ncbi.nlm.nih.gov/pmc/articles/PMC6806981/

Velardi, A. M., Anoldo, P., Nigro, S., & Navarra, G. (2024). Advancements in Bariatric Surgery: A comparative review of laparoscopic and robotic techniques. *Journal of Personalized Medicine, 14*(2), 151. https://doi.org/10.3390/jpm14020151

Abeles, D., & Shikora, S. A. (2008). Bariatric surgery: Current concepts and future directions. *Aesthetic Surgery Journal, 28*(1), 79–84. https://doi.org/10.1016/j.asj.2007.09.007

Sall, A. R., & Jones, M. W. (2023, July 8). *Bariatric surgery preoperative assessment.* StatPearls - NCBI Bookshelf. https://www.ncbi.nlm.nih.gov/books/NBK594256/

UCSF Health. (2024, April 5). *Life after bariatric surgery.* ucsfhealth.org. https://www.ucsfhealth.org/education/life-after-bariatric-surgery#:~:text=Your%20daily%20caloric%20intake%20should,low%20in%20carbohydrates%20and%20sugars.

AdventHealth. (2023, March 9). *4 ways to get mentally ready for bariatric surgery.* https://www.adventhealth.com/blog/4-ways-get-mentally-ready-bariatric-surgery#:~:text=Build%20Coping%20Skills,other%20coping%20strategies%20before%20surgery.

Bariatric surgery - Mayo Clinic. (2023c, October 18).

https://www.mayoclinic.org/tests-procedures/bariatric-surgery/about/pac-20394258#:~:text=This%20is%20a%20two%2Dpart,small%20intestine%2C%20called%20the%20duodenum.

Recovery from Bariatric Surgery - Advanced Surgical Associates. (n.d.). https://www.atlantichealth.org/locations/atlantic-medical-group/advanced-surgical-associates/weight-loss-surgery/recovery.html#:~:text=Your%20hospital%20stay%20will%20vary,bypass%3B%20usually%20stay%20two%20nights.

UCSF Health. (2023, May 8). *Recovering from Bariatric Surgery*. ucsfhealth.org. https://www.ucsfhealth.org/education/recovering-from-bariatric-surgery#:~:text=After%20surgery%2C%20you%20need%20to,dedication%20to%20this%20multifaceted%20plan.

Jefftormey. (2024, February 23). *Mood swings after bariatric surgery: What to expect*. Lenox Hill Bariatric Surgery Program, Manhattan NY. https://www.nycbariatrics.com/blog/understanding-mood-swings-after-bariatric-surgery/#:~:text=Patients%20experiencing%20mood%20changes%20after,feelings%20can%20be%20incredibly%20helpful.

Davis, A. (2018, October 10). *Early and late complications of bariatric operation*. https://www.ncbi.nlm.nih.gov/pmc/articles/PMC6203132/.

Dumping syndrome after gastric bypass surgery. (2024, April 26). Johns Hopkins Medicine. https://www.hopkinsmedicine.org/health/wellness-and-prevention/dumping-syndrome-after-gastric-bypass-surgery#:~:text=What%20is%20dumping%20syndrome%20after,30%20minutes%20after%20a%20meal.

Keshishian, A. (2020, March 28). *Coping Skills after Bariatric Surgery*. DSSurgery. https://www.dssurgery.com/coping-skills-after-bariatric-surgery/

Transformation: After Bariatric Surgery Recovery & Support | WDH. (n.d.). https://www.wdhospital.org/wdh/services-and-specialties/weight-management-weight-loss-surgery/transformation-after-bariatric-surgery

Managing Weight Regain after Bariatric Surgery. (n.d.). https://www.texashealth.org/Health-and-Wellness/Bariatrics/Managing-Weight-Regain-after-Bariatric-Surgery#:~:text=Schedule%20regular%20visits%20with%20your,regular%20diet%20in%20smaller%20amounts.

https://chatgpt.com

About the Author

With over 19 years of rich and diverse experience, Dominic has established himself as a distinguished Educational Consultant and Business Development Executive. Renowned for his flexibility and adaptability, Dominic thrives in agile and highly competitive environments, consistently driving success and innovation.

Throughout his extensive career, Dominic has demonstrated exceptional communication and organizational skills, significantly contributing to the continuous improvement of the organizations he has been a part of. His ability to seamlessly adapt to new procedures and dynamic business environments has been instrumental in navigating the complexities of the publishing industry.

Dominic's profound understanding of educational content and market dynamics positions him as a forward-thinking leader, adept at identifying opportunities and implementing strategic initiatives that foster growth and development. His commitment to excellence and passion for delivering high-quality educational materials make him a valuable asset in the world of publishing.

You can connect with me on:
🐦 https://x.com/singh_domi87960
📘 https://www.facebook.com/dominic.ajithsingh

www.ingramcontent.com/pod-product-compliance
Lightning Source LLC
Chambersburg PA
CBHW051839250726
48659CB00005B/1922